101 Comforting Things to Do

WHILE YOU'RE GETTING BETTER
AT HOME OR IN THE HOSPITAL

ERICA LEVY KLEIN

101 Comforting Things to Do While You're Getting Better At Home or in the Hospital
© 1998 by Erica Levy Klein.

Library of Congress Cataloging-in-Publication Data

Klein, Erica Levy
101 Comforting Things to Do While You're Getting Better / by Erica Levy Klein

      p.   cm.

Includes index.

ISBN 1-56561-132-2; $8.95

Edited by: Jolene Steffer
Cover Design: Claire Lewis
Art/Production Manager: Claire Lewis
Text Design & Production: David Enyeart

10   9   8   7   6   5   4   3   2   1

$\mathcal{C}$ONTENTS ✦ ✦ ✦

For three people who illuminated the journey:
Madge Treeger, Jean Chase, and David Levy

ACKNOWLEDGMENTS ✦ ✦ ✦

I'd like to extend my heartfelt thanks to all of the authors, publishers, organizations, cartoon syndicates, and magazines that allowed me to use the material included in this book. They are listed individually with each excerpt. My deepest gratitude also to Cheryl Kimball, Chronimed's Director of Publishing, who believed in this book enough to give it a second chance. And to my former husband and present friend, Ken Kroll, who provided encouragement, support, and transportation during the countless late nights and still earlier mornings that resulted in this book.

$\mathcal{A}$BOUT THE INFORMATION IN THIS BOOK ✦ ✦ ✦

Although *101 Comforting Things to Do While You're Getting Better* is an "information celebration" that draws from many reputable sources, it is not meant to substitute for professional advice from your health care provider. Our litigious society being what it is, if you choose to follow any of the advice in this book, you do so at your own initiative.

Also, please note that information about the availability or pricing of certain items or services may be subject to change even though the facts were carefully checked before publication.

Please write to me at the following address if you discover any of the information in this book is no longer current, or if you have suggestions of your own. I always welcome your thoughts and comments.

Erica Levy Klein
c/o Chronimed Publishing
10900 Red Circle Drive
Minnetonka, MN 55343

$\mathcal{F}$OREWORD ✦ ✦ ✦

As a physician I am constantly reminded about how important it is for someone ill or injured to experience what I call a "quality recuperation." In the many cases I've observed, the positive nature of the recuperation and the degree to which the patient felt in control of his or her situation played a key role in their steady progress and their return to good health.

Even when patients were dealing with chronic pain or a terminal illness, the way they spent their hours in the hospital or at home made a tremendous difference in how they lived their lives and how they related to others.

Whenever I think of how much a quality recuperation can mean to someone, I remember Sarah, a 56-year-old woman admitted to the hospital with a heart attack complicated by pneumonia. After bypass surgery and six weeks of intensive high-tech medical care, I was finally able to send Sarah home with an excellent prognosis. Naturally, I thought she'd be delighted, but as an attendant wheeled her to her son's waiting car, she seemed overwhelmingly sad. I asked her what was wrong, and she told me, "I feel like I've been here for six years instead of six weeks. Every minute seemed like an hour."

I subsequently learned that Sarah's feelings are more the rule than the exception. And it's not surprising. Whenever you take independent people, accustomed to daily interactions with family, friends, or associates, and suddenly move them to a setting where the entire focus is on what's wrong with them—a setting where they have very little else to distract them—you can virtually guarantee they will suffer from boredom, depression, or both.

In Sarah's case, there was very little to occupy her time other than occasional family visits, deciding what to order for her next meal, and watching television, and although I once suggested some novels, she frequently felt too ill to concentrate for even a short time.

That's why I'm so pleased that Erica Levy Klein has chosen to write *101 Comforting Things to Do While You're Getting Better.* I am certain that this brief, friendly book will contribute to the healing process of any patient, at any stage of recuperation.

The author describes many proven techniques for lessening pain, eliminating boredom, and dealing with the sadness that inevitably affects anyone who has ever suffered from a serious medical problem. I believe if a patient tries some of these activities and coping methods, he or she can avoid many common pitfalls of the medical world and return to complete health far more quickly.

I am hopeful this book will be made available to anyone who faces a medical problem that requires recuperation in a hospital, at home, or in an extended care facility or nursing home. As a physician, I welcome any new approach that supports the healing process, and I cannot think of a more important one than *101 Comforting Things to Do While You're Getting Better.*

John Daniels, MD
Associate Clinical Professor
Washington University School
of Medicine

$\mathcal{I}$NTRODUCTION ✦ ✦ ✦

A Few Words From a Caring Friend

Even in today's world of medical miracles, recuperating from an illness, accident, or surgery can be a surprisingly difficult and lonely process. Not only can progress seem maddeningly slow, but boredom and pain often remind you that you are physically vulnerable and temporarily powerless.

This book was written to lessen those unpleasant feelings, to empower you as much as possible, and to comfort you at a time in your life when you may be feeling anywhere from slightly "out of it" to completely incapacitated. Having been a hospital patient myself and having helped friends and loved ones through the same process, I have very few unrealistic expectations about what you will be able to accomplish using a paperback book as your one and only guide to faster healing.

But I still cherish the hope that *101 Comforting Things to Do While You're Getting Better* will be able to do what a loving friend or family member would do—hold your hand, distract you, amuse you, and help you cope with all the aspects of being "on the mend" in a hospital, nursing home, convalescent center, or even in your own home.

Which brings us to why this book is such a shameless hodgepodge of inspiration and information, suggestions and tips, factoids, diversions, and amusements. It's because I fully intend for it to be the first-ever "comfort book" for the indisposed—a grown-up, connect-the-dots book for the adult set.

You'll find the information presented here in dozens of easy-to-digest small sections so you don't have to wade through lots of pages when all you want to do is make it to the next pain pill or to the next round of visiting hours. And you'll not only discover how to cope with pain and discomfort a little better but also get lots of tips on proven "boredom busters"—those diversions and activities that tend to make the hours fly by when all the minutes seem to do is crawl.

I hope you'll find *101 Comforting Things to Do While You're Getting Better* both helpful and hopeful. In the meantime, I'll simply close by saying a heartfelt prayer for your speedy recovery and your complete return to good health.

Erica Levy Klein
January 1998

Nature, time, and patience are the three great physicians.
—Henry George Bohn

part one

BANISHING BOREDOM

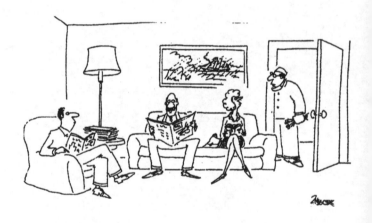

"O.K. Who else needs an operation before I put this stuff away?"

Sweet Nothings

Give yourself permission to do nothing and not feel guilty about it. The world would be a much better place if more people did nothing now and then, don't you agree? Just think of all the messes that might never have been made, to say nothing of wars. Doing nothing also conserves energy. It doesn't cost anything. It's even non-fattening.

From *The Fine Art of Recuperation: Surviving and Thriving After Illness, Accident and Surgery,* by Regina Sara Ryan. © 1989, renewed 1997. Used with permission. For information contact: Hohm Press, PO Box 2501, Prescott, AZ 86302. 1-800-381-2700.

Lighten Up

Generally, it's not advisable to try heavy reading while you're still in the hospital. Keep the world's problems off your back for as long as you can. Even reading the newspaper or watching the TV news may expose you to more bad news than you want. Experiment with remaining uninformed for a few days at a time, and learn what that does for your spirits. When wounded in any way, you're more susceptible to depressing news than you would be if you were stronger.

From *The Fine Art of Recuperation: Surviving and Thriving After Illness, Accident and Surgery,* by Regina Sara Ryan. © 1989, renewed 1997. Used with permission. For information contact: Hohm Press, PO Box 2501, Prescott, AZ 86302. 1-800-381-2700.

ℬooks to Go

Many books can help you as you heal. Some will help you pass the
time; others will assist with specific problems. Still others will be like
old friends, just keeping you company. If you can't get to a library or
bookstore, you may still be only a phone call away from getting the
books you need. Take advantage of the services offered by many
libraries. Often they have a volunteer or homebound program that
provides home delivery of the books you want. Call your local branch
for information. Bookstores will often ship an order directly to your
hospital room or charge your purchase (plus shipping) over the
phone. So call and inquire.

From *The Fine Art of Recuperation: Surviving and Thriving After Illness, Accident
and Surgery,* by Regina Sara Ryan. © 1989, renewed 1997. Used with permission.
For information contact: Hohm Press, PO Box 2501, Prescott, AZ 86302.
1-800-381-2700.

Reading Matters

Here are some suggestions for keeping yourself occupied with interesting reading that can help make even the dullest recuperation more interesting:

✧ Read every book by one author: every spy novel, every romance, etc.

✧ Read every book in a series, fiction or nonfiction.

✧ If you like mystery novels, switch to science fiction.

✧ Read biographies of great people and famous villains.

✧ Read books that will help your career.

✧ Reread your old textbooks. Remember how to do geometry? Or borrow your children's or grandchildren's textbooks.

❖ Read a road atlas. Take a mental vacation—plotting a trip across the West on Route 66, or figuring out how long it would take to drive to Orlando, Florida. Trace the names of towns across the country as the land was gradually settled.

❖ Read all the sections of the newspaper. Get a different newspaper delivered. Or ask your friends to recycle their newspapers and magazines at your home.

❖ Subscribe to newsletters published by associations.

❖ Read recipes or cookbooks.

❖ Read joke books. Learn knock-knock jokes or elephant jokes, or read cartoon books.

Surfing to Wellness

If you own a laptop computer or if you can borrow or rent one, keep it handy by your bedside to check out this helpful Internet site for health-related information:

✧ http://www.lycos.com/health/

The following site is a good source for mental health information:

✧ http://www.cmhc.com/

*B*right *S*pots

Experienced "bed-liers" will tell you that adding a bit of color or aliveness to yourself or your immediate environment will go a long way in helping to brighten your spirits. Use green plants or other living things—a bird in a cage, an aquarium of fish, etc. Try varying the light in the room by removing curtains or changing light bulbs. Ask a friend to hang a new poster or picture on your wall. The possibilities for banishing boredom are endless.

From *The Fine Art of Recuperation: Surviving and Thriving After Illness, Accident and Surgery,* by Regina Sara Ryan. © 1989, renewed 1997. Used with permission. For information contact: Hohm Press, PO Box 2501, Prescott, AZ 86302. 1-800-381-2700.

Cheerful Scents

Incense, if used sparingly, can totally change the environment for the better, especially if your room tends to smell "sickly." Room fresheners are available at all grocery stores. Or how about putting a drop or two of scented oil on the light bulbs?

Catalog Avalanche

If you think now is a good time to get more catalogs arriving in your mailbox, a great shortcut is *The Catalog Handbook,* a quarterly publication that lists more than 5,000 catalogs by category and alphabetically. From "Aircraft Accessories" and "Antiques" to "Woodworking Supplies" and "Yarns," this handy resource has a catalog for every interest under the sun and tells you how to get on the mailing list.

The Catalog Handbook is available for $7.99 per copy or $27.99 per year, including postage. Call (414) 272-9977 or write to: Enterprise Magazines, 1020 North Broadway, Suite 111, Milwaukee, WI 53202.

Bedside Travel

One of the best travel gadget resources in the world is *Magellan's Catalog*, (800) 962-4943. It's crammed with things that can help the time go faster, including language learning aids such as cassette tapes, phrase books, and nifty pocket translators that do things like turn any English phrase into Japanese and vice versa.

Fantasy Hotels

It only costs $15 to experience some of the world's most luxurious hotels and sumptuous resorts when you send for *Resorts and Great Hotels: The International Guide to the World's Best.* It's a delightful inch-thick magazine that lets you travel in style even when you can't get out of bed! For credit card orders, call (805) 687-1422.

Learning Curve

Now is a great time to make a list of 10 activities you always (or almost always) wanted to do but were afraid to try. Consider things you'd like to build, skills you'd like to acquire, knowledge you'd like to gain, creative ideas you've always wanted to express yourself, or social activities you've always wanted to enjoy.

Now look over your list and narrow it down to three. You might pick the three that seem the least threatening or the ones that provide the greatest challenge. It's up to you! To make your goal a reality, you can use one or all of these five methods:

✧ Try to learn all by yourself, even though this may involve some trial and error.

✧ Hire an expert to teach you, or barter for their services.

✧ Find a class at a local high school, YMCA or YWCA, university, or community college. A benefit to this approach is that you'll have the camaraderie of other students and the structure of a class to support and pace your learning.

✧ Audio- or videotapes.

✧ Friends or relatives.

From *Healing the Body Betrayed: A Self-Paced, Self-Help Guide to Regaining Psychological Control of Your Chronic Illness,* by Robert A. Klein, PhD, and Marcia Goodman Landau, PhD © 1992. Chronimed Publishing, Minneapolis, MN $12.95.

Sense-O-Rama

Check off any of the sensory activities below that you can associate
with a happy memory or childhood pleasure. Think of ways you
might be able to re-experience that sensation.

SIGHTS

candles	crowds
mirrors	the moon
handsome men/pretty women	color
clouds	photos
luxury autos	

SOUNDS
music

crickets

tuned auto engine

cat purring

children playing

pleasant voices

fizz of a soda can

rain

ice cubes tinkling

SMELLS
food

gasoline

leather

air after rainfall

flowers

cut grass

clean sheets

sweat

From *Healing the Body Betrayed: A Self-Paced, Self-Help Guide to Regaining Psychological Control of Your Chronic Illness,* by Robert A. Klein, PhD, and Marcia Goodman Landau, PhD © 1992. Chronimed Publishing, Minneapolis, MN $12.95.

Band-Aids for Boredom

Think of 10 restaurants you've eaten in where you've enjoyed wonderful food or memorable experiences. Try to remember what you ate, what the interior looked like, and who you were with.

From *The Fine Art of Recuperation: Surviving and Thriving After Illness, Accident and Surgery,* by Regina Sara Ryan. © 1989, renewed 1997. Used with permission. For information contact: Hohm Press, PO Box 2501, Prescott, AZ 86302. 1-800-381-2700.

*P*ersonal *I*ntroductions

If you're really stuck for something to read, why not take a few minutes to thoroughly review your admission packet? While not the most scintillating reading in the world, this packet is filled with useful information about everything from walking privileges and chapel services to visiting hours and overnight accommodations for your visitors.

It's a Draw!

On one side of a blank piece of paper, draw yourself as you feel now. On the other side, draw yourself as you will be when you are fully well. Feel free to portray yourself in an abstract form.

Draw your illness or accident. Again, be abstract. Draw the healing agents that are eliminating the illness or accident. Show the interaction between them.

Draw any feeling you are currently enduring: fear, doubt, guilt, etc.

Draw an ally—a friend, angel, animal, or symbol.

Draw laughter, hilarity, silliness, or absurdity.

Draw a fantasy place of comfort and safety.

From *The Fine Art of Recuperation: Surviving and Thriving After Illness, Accident and Surgery*, by Regina Sara Ryan. © 1989, renewed 1997. Used with permission. For information contact: Hohm Press, PO Box 2501, Prescott, AZ 86302. 1-800-381-2700.

Writing Out Recuperation

✧ Tell the story of your illness or accident. Start at the beginning and record everything you know about it. Do this again in a week and see if your outlook is different in the two stories.

✧ Have a dialogue with your illness, a part of your body, or another part of your mind. Ask it about the crisis you are experiencing, why it is happening now, and what it has to teach you. Be candid.

✧ Start a conversation with a wise teacher, a spiritual leader, a famous doctor, or anyone else who can help you in your recuperation. Communicate your deepest feelings, your needs, and your fears. Then write a reply to yourself. Give yourself healing advice.

From *The Fine Art of Recuperation: Surviving and Thriving After Illness, Accident and Surgery*, by Regina Sara Ryan. © 1989, renewed 1997. Used with permission. For information contact: Hohm Press, PO Box 2501, Prescott, AZ 86302. 1-800-381-2700.

Look Better, Feel Better

Here are a few ways to enhance your body image, lift your spirits, and make good use of your time as you recuperate:

✧ Get a haircut or change the style. Even asking a friend to simply wash and dry your hair will provide a welcome change.

✧ Get a manicure or pedicure.

✧ Get a foot massage.

✧ Attend to your teeth and gums.

✧ Wear warm, lively, or tranquil colors to suit your moods. Choose colors that bring out a healthy glow in your skin tone.

✧ Dress for energy in a jogging suit and bright shirt rather than crumpled pajamas. Or put on an attractive nightgown or nightshirt.

✧ Do facial exercises to soften lines and tone muscles.

✧ Give yourself a facial massage. Knead, slap, stroke, and roll the skin on your face (gently around the eyes). Consider that you're trying to wake up all the cells and increase circulation throughout the face.

✧ If your doctor says it's OK, treat your skin to a moisturizing lotion or cream, or even an oil treatment.

✧ Try something just for fun. Try repainting your cast, putting on a hat or brightly colored scarf, or adding a temporary tattoo to a place where only the doctor will find it. One man donned a gorilla mask whenever he expected yet another somber visitor.

From *The Fine Art of Recuperation: Surviving and Thriving After Illness, Accident and Surgery,* by Regina Sara Ryan. © 1989, renewed 1997. Used with permission. For information contact: Hohm Press, PO Box 2501, Prescott, AZ 86302. 1-800-381-2700.

Moving Onward and Upward

Simple isometric exercises like the ones below will help you maintain and increase your range of motion. However, always consult your physician before undertaking any exercise during recuperation. While lying down and looking straight ahead, do the following:

✧ Place the heel of your hand on your forehead and push your forehead against your hand.

✧ Place the palm of your hand against the back of your head, and push your head backward against the force of your hand.

✧ Place the palm of your right hand against the right side of your head and push your head sideward, resisting the pressure of your hand. Do the same for your left side.

✧ Clench your teeth, raise your head slightly, and forcefully pull the corners of your mouth outward and down.

While in a sitting position:

✧ Put the palms of your hands together and forcefully push them
   toward each other.

✧ Clasp your hands together and then try to forcefully pull them
   apart.

From *I Can Cope,* by Judith L. Johnson, RN, PhD, and Linda Klein. © 1994.
Chronimed Publishing, Minneapolis, MN $12.95.

Tours and Detours

Some hospitals have a special lounge area for patients or a veranda for good-weather days. Go there for a change of scene. Go to these places with your visitors so they don't have to see you in bed. Sit in these havens to think, read (the light is probably better there, too), or even nap. For an hour or so you can put aside the fact you are in a hospital.

If yourhospital has no sitting area for patients, get up and walk around anyway (assuming you have your doctor's permission). When you get out of bed and step out of your room, you not only improve you constitution, you also issue a clear declaration of independence.

From *Take This Book to the Hospital with You,* by Charles B. Inlander and Ed Weiner. ©1985, 1991 by People's Medical Society. Reprinted by permission of Pantheon Books, a division of Random House, Inc.

*B*edtime *S*tory

If you're recuperating at home, make your bed as colorful and sensu-
ous as possible. Give special attention to the colors and textures of
bedding. If you have never used cotton flannel sheets, treat yourself.
Comfortable even in the warmest weather, they provide a nurturing,
soothing feeling.

From *The Fine Art of Recuperation: Surviving and Thriving After Illness, Accident
and Surgery,* by Regina Sara Ryan. © 1989, renewed 1997. Used with permission.
For information contact: Hohm Press, PO Box 2501, Prescott, AZ 86302.
1-800-381-2700.

𝒯𝒱 or 𝒩ot 𝒯𝒱? 𝒯hat 𝒥s the 𝒬uestion

Ask yourself these three questions:

✧ Am I laughing more as a result of what I see on TV?

✧ Do I feel better about myself or about life in general as a result of watching TV?

✧ Does my pain or self-focus diminish as I watch TV?

If you can answer yes to any of the above, you are probably using TV wisely. But if you answered no, you may want to consider activities.

From *The Fine Art of Recuperation: Surviving and Thriving After Illness, Accident and Surgery,* by Regina Sara Ryan. © 1989, renewed 1997. Used with permission. For information contact: Hohm Press, PO Box 2501, Prescott, AZ 86302. 1-800-381-2700.

Approaching Avoidance

Sometimes being clear about what you don't want inspires you to know better what you do want. Make a list of all the ways you definitely do not wish to spend your time. Staring out the window, talking about someone's uninteresting relative, or watching TV reruns is a good start.

From *The Fine Art of Recuperation: Surviving and Thriving After Illness, Accident and Surgery,* by Regina Sara Ryan. © 1989, renewed 1997. Used with permission. For information contact: Hohm Press, PO Box 2501, Prescott, AZ 86302. 1-800-381-2700.

𝒲orking on ℒeisure

Force yourself to get back in the swing of leisure activities as soon as possible. Can't think of what you'd like to do? Here are some suggestions:

✧ Take a walk and reacquaint yourself with a favorite area or park

✧ Put in a new bush or nurture a new plant.

✧ Cook a gourmet dinner from recipes in a magazine.

✧ Collect stamps or rocks.

✧ Sew a new outfit or work on a craft project.

✧ Take in a movie.

✧ Visit an old friend.

✧ Join a new club.

From *I Can Cope,* by Judith L. Johnson, RN, PhD, and Linda Klein. © 1994. Chronimed Publishing, Minneapolis, MN $12.95.

part two

ENTERTAINMENT,
AMUSEMENTS,
AND DIVERSIONS

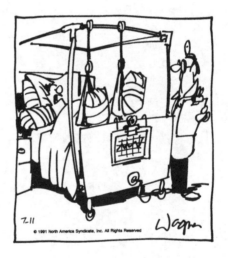

"Will I be able to play golf Saturday?"

Reprinted with special permission of North America Syndicate. © 1991.

Wearable Massage

These days, a good massage comes in many other forms besides a massage therapist. You can find vibrating collars, pillows, and foot stools at most major department stores, local gadget stores, or by mail order.

No-Hassle Gardening

A good low-maintenance project when you're recuperating is an herb garden featuring your favorite culinary herbs and spices. An herb garden can give you a tremendous sense of peace and hope as you watch it progress. It's easiest if you start with seedlings, as opposed to seeds. Just keep your herbs in a sunny window, and don't forget to water them once or twice a week.

Video Visits

Why wait until you have enough money to take the trip of your dreams? The free *International Video Network Video Catalog* (800-669-4486) can take you there for the price of just a videotape.

You can explore castles, churches, shops, and shrines amidst the charm of Europe's most romantic cities. Wander among streams, rivers, picturesque villages, and the ruins of ancient civilizations in South America. Discover the mysteries of the Orient and marvel at the natural wonders of the United States, the wildlife of Africa, and the charms of the Caribbean. It's all waiting for you to explore!

Hobbies on Parade

Hobbies can be great fun and also lifesavers when you are confined for a while. Choose a few topics that grab you. Then consider what you can do to begin your exploration. Call your library or local college for references on the topic. Or ask family members and friends for books, Web sites, or tapes on the subject:

antiques	economics
archeology	embroidery
architecture	fishing
art	flower arranging
astronomy	flying
auto maintenance	food preservation
backgammon	foreign languages
basket weaving	furniture design
batik	gardening

biology

bonsai

bridge

calligraphy

carpentry

cartooning

ceramics

chamber music

chess

coin collecting

collages

computers

crocheting

doll collecting

drawing

model building

mythology

gemstones

genealogy

geography

geology

history

home repair

hypnotism

indoor plants

investing

jazz

juggling

landscaping

literature

magic

math

real estate

recipes

needlepoint
opera
origami
painting
philosophy
physics
play writing
pottery
psychology
quilting

robotics
sailing
Shakespeare
stained glass
stamp collecting
travel/adventure
weaving
wine making
yoga

Noteworthy Thoughts

If you just don't feel like writing your thoughts down, there are pocket dictation machines that will allow you to record several hours of ideas, thoughts, and reminders without putting pen to paper. The voice activated recording (VAR) capability starts the recorder only when you speak so you don't waste tape while you're thinking. And they usually run for five hours or more on a single AAA battery.

𝒥apping into 𝒥apes

If you have difficulty reading, holding a book, or focusing your attention, books on tape are a godsend. Call your local public library to find out if it carries any, or inquire at a well-stocked bookstore in your area. Or try the following:

Books on Tape, P.O. Box 7900, Newport Beach, CA 92658. Will ship anywhere in the United States. Tapes can be rented or purchased. To order tapes or a catalog, call (800) 626-3333.

Audio Renaissance Tapes, 9110 Sunset Blvd., Suite 200, Los Angeles, CA 90069. (213) 273-9755. A fine selection of interesting and useful tapes, including *Getting Well* by Dr. O. Carl Simonton, as well as others by well-known authors in the field of health and well-being.

Dove Audio, 301 North Canon Drive, Suite 203, Beverly Hills, CA 90210. (800) 328-DOVE or (800) 345-9945. Lots of romances, current best-sellers, sci-fi, celebrity biographies, and humor.

Tattered Cover Bookstore, Denver, CO. (800) 833-2327. In Colorado, call (800) 821-2896.

Dial - a - Distraction

Look in the business section of the white pages of your phone directory under "Dial-A..." to find numbers for inspiring and interesting messages. Call, listen, and let your mind drift away. Just be sure to steer clear of any numbers that may indicate a charge, such as those with 900- prefixes.

From *The Fine Art of Recuperation: Surviving and Thriving After Illness, Accident and Surgery,* by Regina Sara Ryan. © 1989, renewed 1997. Used with permission. For information contact: Hohm Press, PO Box 2501, Prescott, AZ 86302. 1-800-381-2700.

Best of the Worst

Compose your own "Bests" or "Worsts" list, including answers to such questions as: What was the worst movie you ever saw? What was your best vacation? Who is your worst-dressed family member? What was the worst meal you ever had on Thanksgiving? And so on.

Stress-Busting Sounds

Check your local music or book store for the Environments series or Solitude series of nature sounds on cassette or CD. There is also a full line of soothing videos available. Or you can order them directly by calling Backroads Distributors at (800) 825-4848 or writing them at 417 Tamal Plaza, Corte Madera, CA 94925.

.

From *The Fine Art of Recuperation: Surviving and Thriving After Illness, Accident and Surgery*, by Regina Sara Ryan. © 1989, renewed 1997. Used with permission. For information contact: Hohm Press, PO Box 2501, Prescott, AZ 86302. 1-800-381-2700.

Classic Remedies

❖ Bach, Double Concerto or Violin Concertos 1 and 2; Brandenburg Concertos.

❖ Mozart, Violin Concertos 3 and 5.

❖ Pachelbel's Canon/Baroque Favorites.

❖ Chopin, Nocturnes.

❖ Beethoven, Symphony No. 6 (the Pastoral).

❖ Dvořák, Cello Concerto, and Tchaikovsky, Rococo Variations.

❖ Mendelssohn, Violin Concertos.

From *The Fine Art of Recuperation: Surviving and Thriving After Illness, Accident and Surgery,* by Regina Sara Ryan. © 1989, renewed 1997. Used with permission. For information contact: Hohm Press, PO Box 2501, Prescott, AZ 86302. 1-800-381-2700.

Kooshy Kooshy Koo

My favorite personal stress-buster is a Koosh Ball, a snuggly porcupine-like ball with soft, rubbery bristles that makes it hard to put down. Throw it, roll it, or just hold it and be comforted by it. Koosh Balls are available in large or small sizes or in animal shapes at most toy stores. And don't overlook the Koosh Ball's highly popular animal cousins, Beanie Babies.

24-Hour Stress Soother

Many hospitals, HMOs, and insurance providers now offer recordings on a variety of medical and psychological subjects that are accessible by phone around the clock. Check with the community education department of your hospital or call your insurer. In the New York City area, Lenox Hill Hospital offers stress-reducing messages through its Tel-Med service at (212) 434-3200.

Fifteen Quick Exercises

Exercise can relax you, improve your circulation, help with lung expansion, and improve sleep. Get your doctor's permission first, then start slowly and easily.

Each of the following exercises is meant to be done individually:

1. Put your hands on the chair arms or in your lap. Pull your shoulder blades together while you breathe in deeply. Relax and slowly breathe out.

2. Shrug your shoulders up and slowly let them down. Then completely relax.

3. Place your hands on the arms or seat of a chair. Push with your hands as if to lift yourself out of the chair. Do not push with your feet.

4. Squeeze your buttocks tightly together. Count to 5. Then relax. Don't hold your breath.

5. Put your right hand on your left knee and try to lift your knee up, but press so hard with your hand that you can't relax. Relax. Repeat with your other leg.

6. Lift one arm in front of you, then up over your head, keeping your elbow straight. Repeat with the other arm. If this is comfortable, do both arms together and reach for the ceiling.

7. Lift one arm to the side and over your head, keeping your elbow straight. Repeat with the other arm. If this is comfortable, do both together and reach for the ceiling.

8. Straighten your knees as much as possible, one at a time. Then do both.

9. Press your heels into the floor as if to lift yourself out of your chair.

10. Dig your heels into the floor as if to dig a hole.

11. Place your hands on your shoulders. Rotate your elbows in circles.

12. Cross your arms in front of your chest. Then gently bring them back as if to touch your elbows behind your back.

13. Put your hands together in front of your chest. Straighten your fingers as much as possible. Push hands together. Relax.

14. Fold your hands together. Try to pull them apart.

15. Lift your foot slightly off the floor. Point your toes and foot up and down. Then make circles with your foot.

From *I Can Cope,* by Judith L. Johnson, RN, PhD, and Linda Klein. © 1994. Chronimed Publishing, Minneapolis, MN $12.95.

Crossword Secrets

These are inside tips from Stanley Newman, one of America's most prolific puzzle makers and editors and a world-class puzzle solver.

1. Don't automatically start with 1 Across. The best answer to put in a puzzle first is the one you're sure of. Most of the time, a "fill-in-the-blank" clue is a good place to start.

2. After you've written the first answer, try to fill in answers that already have one or more letters filled in from crossing words. It's almost always easier to figure out.

3. Don't jump around, filling in answers all over the puzzle. Your solving will be easier and faster if you concentrate on one area of the puzzle at a time. If you're unable to fill in any answers in the area you're working in, look for a fill-in-the-blank clue in a nearby section of the puzzle and try to link up with the area you were working on before.

4. If you become hopelessly stuck, it's OK to take a peek at the answers for a little help. Some people think it's cheating, but it's perfectly all right. You won't get stuck on the same clues next time if you learn them now.

5. When you're done, check your answers with the printed solution. You'd be surprised how often an answer you thought was right isn't.

6. Don't solve puzzles in pen unless you never make mistakes. If you want to impress onlookers, use an erasable pen.

7. Be choosy about which crosswords you do. Experts agree that the best crosswords are those that contain a broad spectrum of facts (not just dictionary definitions), have lively language, make use of humor and wordplay, and avoid obscure words.

8. Part of the fun of crossword solving comes from getting to know the personalities of the people that create them. For this reason, you should avoid puzzles (in magazines, books, and newspapers) where the author's name is not given.

9. Try to do puzzles that are slightly above your current level of expertise. It's no great accomplishment to fill in a puzzle as fast as you can write if you're not learning anything in the process.

10. Be sure to look up all unfamiliar words and references. This may involve more than your unabridged dictionary, since today's best puzzles use a wide variety of information. But your vocabulary and knowledge base will increase steadily as a result, and that's the best way to improve your solving skill.

From *Inspector Cross Twenty Unique Crossword Capers & Mystery Word Teasers, Volume I,* by Stanley Newman. Lombard Marketing $12.95. (800) 874-6556. *Volume II* is also available from the same company.

Puzzling Newsletters

If you're a true crossword fanatic, you may want to invest in one of these newsletters for puzzle lovers:

Tough Puzzles/$25 for 6 issues
American Crossword Federation
Box 69
Massapequa Park, NY 11762
(516) 795-8823

Puzzleletter/$12 year
Dartnell Cambridge Associates
164 Canal St.
Boston, MA 02114
(617) 723-5969

Healthy Curiosity

One of the things you can do while lying flat on your back is to satisfy your healthy curiosity about the world around you. And two terrific series of books can help:

The first series includes the books *How Do They Do That*, which explores the wonders of today's modern world, and *How Did They Do That*, which takes on mysteries of the far and recent past. These softcover books are $9 each.

The second series, called *Amazing Explanations*, includes three books by David Feldman: *Why Do Clocks Run Clockwise?*, *Who Put the Butter in the Butterfly?*, and *When Do Fish Sleep?* These softcover books are $9 to $10 each. All these books are available at most libraries and bookstores.

Video Voyages

In an effort to provide better patient education about preventive care, as well as certain medical procedures, some hospitals make a selection of videos available to you on a special TV channel. Topics range from Low Back Pain and Osteoporosis to A Day Away From Stress, which offers a welcome 26-minute "vacation" as you follow the steps to relaxation. Screenings are usually held throughout the day, so if you miss one showing, just wait for another one!

Prescription — Laughter

Here are 13 readily available videotapes that can get you laughing…
fast!

1. *Airplane.* A hilarious spoof of the Airport series—and movies in
general. While the jokes don't always work, there are so many of them
that this comedy ends up with enough laughs for three movies.

2. *A Night at the Opera.* Classic Marx Brothers' fare as the brothers go
en masse to the opera. Need I say more?

3. *Animal House.* Still one of the funniest movies ever made. A wild
college fraternity gets placed on "double secret probation" and, of
course, blows it with rock 'n' roll, partying, and general craziness.

4. *The Bank Dick.* W. C. Fields is at his best in this laugh-filled comedy. Fields plays a drunkard who becomes a hero. But the story is just
an excuse for the many moments of hilarity.

5. *Blazing Saddles.* Mel Brooks's raucous spoof of Westerns will have you in stitches, if you aren't already.

6. *Ferris Bueller's Day Off.* The charming tale of a high school legend in his own time who pretends to be ill in order to have a day off from school.

7. *The Goodbye Girl.* Marsha Mason and Richard Dreyfuss are a mismatched pair of New Yorkers forced into becoming roommates in this sparkling Neil Simon classic.

8. *Jay Leno's American Dream.* Comedian and talk show host Jay Leno takes an irreverent look at all that is Americana.

9. *My Man Godfrey.* One of the great screwball comedies of the '30s. William Powell goes from being a hobo to the butler for a wacky family and finds love with Carole Lombard.

10. *Some Like It Hot.* The outlandish story of two men, Jack Lemmon and Tony Curtis, who accidentally witness a gangland slaying and

pose as members of an all-girl band. Marilyn Monroe is at her sensual best as the band's singer.

11. *Trading Places.* An uproarious comedy about what happens when an uptight Philadelphia broker (Dan Aykroyd) and a dynamic, street hustler (Eddie Murphy) change places.

12. *What's Up Doc?* This stars Ryan O'Neal as a studio scientist delightfully led astray by a dizzy Barbra Streisand, who keeps forcing herself into his life. The zany final chase through the streets of San Francisco is one of filmdom's best.

13. *When Harry Met Sally.* Can men and women be friends? This film answers the question by laughing all the way as Billy Crystal and Meg Ryan discover their friendship blooming into romance.

From *The Video Movie Guide,* by Mick Martin and Marsha Porter. © 1998. Ballantine Books, New York, NY. $18.95 (800) 733-3000.

Gambler's Secret

If you consider yourself a gambler, and you'd enjoy playing everything from hand-held poker games to getting expert instruction in casino action and horse racing while you're recuperating, call for a free copy of *The World's Greatest Gaming Catalog*, (800) 345-7017.

part three

UNSTRESS FOR SUCCESS

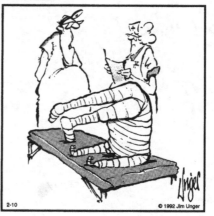

"How's he sleeping at night?"

Relaxing in Place

Some hospital procedures require lying still in uncomfortable positions for a long time. Try these suggestions for relieving the boredom and stress:

✧ Focus on points in the room to provide a diversion.

✧ Daydream about wonderful travel experiences, loving memories, or other pleasant thoughts.

✧ Wiggle your toes or any part of your body you can in a rotating manner.

From *Successful Living with Chronic Illness,* by Kathleen Lewis. © 1989. Avery Publishing Group, Garden City Park, NY $10. To order: (404) 491-6850.

Whiting Out Noise

You know all too well how strange sounds can keep you from getting to sleep in a hospital (or even your home if it's in a noisy neighborhood). Luckily, there are portable "white noise" machines that can unobtrusively fill your room with a wide range of soothing nature sounds—from a light rain to a tropical waterfall. This helpful item is available in many travel gadget stores, or by mail order.

Sick x 2

When an early treatment fails to cure, it doesn't matter why. Whether the treatment was too gentle, the illness too insidious, or the chance of cure too small, the persistence or recurrence of your illness can break your spirit. Recurrence, in particular, can overwhelm you. You feel that you've been twice betrayed: Your body's fallen ill, and then pretended to be cured, only to succumb again to illness.

In illness, as in every other aspect of your life, it's useful to have had some experience. Though no one would choose to be sick in the first place, nor choose to fall sick again and again, the second and subsequent battles with illness, though hard because you're weary, may go well because you're seasoned. If you look to your experience instead of your fatigue, you'll find the means to do what you must do.

From *You Can Make It Back: Coping With Serious Illness,* by Paul M. Levitt and Elissa S. Guralnick. © 1985. Facts on File Publications, New York, NY $16.95. Currently out of print but still available in many libraries. (212) 683-2244.

Breathing Easy

1. Pick a time and place where you won't be disturbed and lie or sit in a comfortable position. If you're in a hospital bed, position the bed at the most comfortable angle or ask a nurse to do this for you.

2. Close your eyes and begin counting backward from 50. Time each count in the following manner to match your breathing. After you exhale, notice that you don't have to breathe in again immediately and can rest comfortably for a few seconds. For some people, this may only be 1 or 2 seconds. For others it may be as long as 20 seconds. Count during this peaceful time when the lungs have paused and the body is still. Count one number for each cycle of breathing in and out.

From *Anxiety, Phobias and Panic: Taking Charge & Conquering Fear,* by Reneau Z. Peurifoy, M.A., M.F.C.C. © 1992. Lifeskills, P.O. Box 7915, Citrus Heights, CA 95621. $12.95. (916) 723-7517.

Comfy Comforters

Whenever I have to face surgery or a hospital stay, I make sure I take either my fuzzy fake chinchilla blanket from home or a quilt that I particularly like. A good resource for down comforters and sheets of every size and shape is *The Company Store* catalog, (800) 323-8000. For dazzling colorful sheets and comforters, try the *Domestications* catalog, (800) 782-7722. And for fake animal-fur throws like my chinchilla, try *A Touch of Class* catalog, (812) 683-3707.

To Treat or Not to Treat

When a treatment is routine or minor, the decision to accept it isn't difficult. But when a treatment will cause sacrifice or pain, offers no guarantee of a cure, causes disfigurement, or subjects you to the risk of lethal side effects, the decision isn't so easy. As you grapple with your choices, compare the probable consequences of accepting treatment with those of refusing it. In particular, after you've consulted with your doctor, take some time to answer these 10 questions:

1. What physical limitations are you likely to face if you are treated and if you are not?

2. Will these limitations be permanent or temporary?

3. What rehabilitation services will be available to you if you're treated and if you're not?

4. How much improvement is rehabilitation likely to achieve?

5. What changes will occur in your self-esteem if you're treated and if you're not?

6. What sexual adjustments will have to be made if you're treated and if you're not?

7. What pleasures and habits will have to be sacrificed if you're treated and if you're not?

8. How will your life or job have to change if you're treated and if you're not?

9. Whose regard are you likely to lose or maintain if you're treated and if you're not?

10. Are you facing a serious threat to your life if you're treated and if you're not?

From *You Can Make It Back: Coping With Serious Illness,* by Paul M. Levitt and Elissa S. Guralnick. © 1985. Facts on File Publications, New York, NY $16.95. Currently out of print but still available in many libraries. (212) 683-2244.

Three Paths Through the Forest

You can react in three different ways to a chronic illness. The first is to give up and forgo any treatment. The second is to deny the diagnosis is true, which leads to despair because you get nowhere. The third road is to get active on your own behalf and take responsibility for your well-being and your goals for the future.

From *Successful Living with Chronic Illness,* by Kathleen Lewis. © 1989. Avery Publishing Group, Garden City Park, NY $10. To order: (404) 491-6850.

Rest Easy

Sleep can be one of the most important healing forces in your life. To ensure you get adequate rest, try not to take your worries to bed with you. If you're plagued by insomnia, remember what pyschologist Dr. David Viscott said in his book *A Natural Sleep*—"You can't solve all your problems at once."

If you still can't sleep, you may want to take the extra step of writing down all your problems and some possible solutions for each one. Your plan of action will help you realize you're not as helpless as you thought and that you don't have to think about your worries all the time.

You Are Not Alone

The first prescription for riding the sometimes frightening or confus-
ing emotional waves that accompany a health crisis is to recognize
that you're not alone in what you're going through. Countless others
have felt this way, too. And while this may not relieve your pain, it
may help to relieve some of your anxiety about it. Truly, nobody else
has ever experienced their crisis in exactly the same way you have. Yet
the reports of many recuperating people about what they felt, what
they feared, and what surprised them are remarkably similar despite
age differences or types of illness.

A Good Cry Is a Good Thing

What do you do if you've identified the reason for the bad feelings, communicated with others about them, sought information, and tried solutions—but nothing helps? This is the time for a good cry. Give in, beat the pillow, throw a few items at the walls (assuming you're at home), and get that tension out of your system. We recommend throwing a light object such as a Nerf ball, since it will give your arm muscles some exercise and won't damage walls or shatter. It may seem absurd to picture yourself throwing sponge balls and sobbing (especially if you're unaccustomed to crying), but nature gave us all the ability to cry for good reasons. A good cry relieves stress and allows you to gather your coping skills once again.

Redefining Yourself

Try not to think of yourself as a sick person. Think of yourself as a healthy person who on this occasion became sick or injured.

From *Healing the Body Betrayed: A Self-Paced, Self-Help Guide to Regaining Psychological Control of Your Chronic Illness,* by Robert A. Klein, Ph D, and Marcia Goodman Landau, PhD © 1992. Chronimed Publishing. Minneapolis, MN $12.95.

*R*emember the *G*uy in the *B*lack *H*at

Take a minute to forgive someone you dislike for his or her many transgressions against you.

Get Angry/Get Hopeful

Both anger and hope are healthy responses to illness. They're expressions of defiance, antidotes to fear and pain, displays of belief in the future. When your weakened body seems a burden fit to be forsaken, anger and hope are the twin engines that keep you moving forward. However, anger can be self-defeating when:

✧ You let yourself sulk and abandon all pleasure until finally it seems you have nothing to live for.

✧ You lash out at others who'd like to be helpful but who finally withdraw out of fear that they merely annoy you.

✧ You cancel your medical appointments or refuse to be treated in order to punish the doctor (or yourself).

✧ You undermine your spirit with constant complaints and fruitless laments.

Even hope, which is so much less threatening, can mock and abuse you if:

✧ You behave unrealistically by engaging, for example, in arduous activities for which you aren't fit.

✧ You trust in blind luck and refuse to be bothered with exercise, diets, and drugs the doctor has ordered.

✧ You grasp at a miracle cure that is proffered by quacks, while spurning a thoroughly safe and effective conventional treatment.

When handled sensibly, anger and hope can protect you from losing respect for yourself. And since self-respect is medicine as strong as a drug, it's a valuable commodity to foster.

From *You Can Make It Back: Coping With Serious Illness,* by Paul M. Levitt and Elissa S. Guralnick. © 1985. Facts on File Publications, New York, NY $16.95. Currently out of print, still available in many libraries. (212) 683-2244.

Practicing Wholeness

Sit in a comfortable chair with your feet on the floor and your arms at your sides. Close your eyes. Breathe in, saying to yourself, "I am…," then breathe out saying, "…relaxed." Continue breathing slowly, silently repeating to yourself something such as, "My hands are…warm; my feet are…warm; my forehead is…cool; my breathing is…deep and smooth; my heartbeat is…calm and steady; I am…happy; I feel calm…and at peace."

From *Coping with Stress,* by the Arthritis Foundation, P.O. Box 19000, Atlanta, GA 30326. Free. (404) 872-7100.

Healthy Goals

For the best mental health, and the greatest emotional maturity, everyone should have a cause, a mission, an aim in life that is constructive and so big that you have to keep on working on it.

From Dr. William C. Menninger, Founder, Menninger Clinic, Topeka, KS.

8 *Steps to Psychological Strength*

1. Choose to make a plan to achieve every day—a written list of simple daily goals that are realistic for you to achieve.

2. Approach others first—be positive.

3. Choose to have fun each day.

4. Choose to see the positive in all things.

5. Choose to be responsible for yourself.

6. Choose to be in the present; don't dwell on the past.

7. Choose to be curious and spontaneous.

8. Choose to be in balance and seek positive responses to stresses.

From *Positive Addiction*, by William Glasser, M.D. © 1988. HarperCollins, New York, NY $10. (212) 207-7000.

Small Blessings

Because a sense of hopefulness can help speed your recuperation, end each day by mentally reviewing the things you're grateful for, no matter how small or insignificant.

Positively Healthy

You can increase your healing potential through the encouraging self-talk known as positive affirmation. Here are some healing affirmations to choose from, or you can use them as a starting point for creating your own:

✧ With every breath, I grow in energy and strength.

✧ My mind, my body, and my soul are all working together to create healing and peace.

✧ I am at peace. I love and accept all of life.

✧ I release the old and welcome the new. Health and happiness are mine.

When composing your own affirmation, steer clear of tentative or negative words like "might," "maybe," "hope," "will be," "don't," "not," or "never." These thoughts will undermine your newfound good feelings.

One for the Road

Focus on even the smallest amount of progress in your recovery. Don't dwell on what still lies ahead of you—think about how far you've come, and allow yourself to savor the comfort of that knowledge.

From Ellen Bern and Barry Mizes, St. Louis, MO.

part four

PAINKICKERS

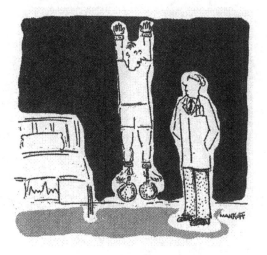

"I think I'd like to explore some treatment alternatives."

Redefining Control

The unpredictability of chronic pain makes it seem we have lost control of our lives. In addition, the standard we may have set for ourselves in our daily lives may no longer be attainable, causing an even greater sense of helplessness. In reality, however, we are still in control of many areas of our lives. And by redirecting our energy toward managing pain, we can experience a higher degree of control in that area as well.

From *How to Beat the Chronic Pain Blues,* by Sandy Plotz. $3. Reprinted with permission of Chronic Pain Outreach of Greater St. Louis, Inc. (314) 768-1350.

12 Steps to More Effective Pain Control

1. Accept the fact that you have pain.

2. Set specific goals for work, hobbies, and social activities toward which you will work.

3. Let yourself get angry with your pain if it seems to be getting the best of you.

4. Take your analgesics on a strict schedule, and then taper off until you're no longer taking any.

5. Get in the best physical shape possible, and keep fit.

6. Learn how to relax, and practice relaxation techniques regularly.

7. Keep yourself busy.

8. Pace your activities.

9. Have family and friends support only your healthy behavior, not your invalidism.

10. Be open and reasonable with your doctor.

11. Practice effective empathy with others having pain problems.

12. Remain hopeful.

Reprinted by permission of The Putnam Publishing Group from *Mastering Pain*, by Richard Sternbach. © 1987 by Richard Sternbach.

Dear Diary

Sometimes it's helpful to keep a diary for the next time you see your doctor. In the diary, be sure to include any activity that increases or decreases your pain. Also, include how frequently you take your pain medication and the amount taken. In addition, note if you use the medication before the pain starts or after you're already in pain. Finally, be sure to assign a number from 1 (no pain) to 10 (the worst pain you can imagine) that best describes your pain.

From *I Can Cope,* by Judith L. Johnson, RN, PhD, and Linda Klein. © 1994. Chronimed Publishing, Minneapolis, MN $12.95.

A-d-a-p-t

If you're feeling truly overwhelmed by pain, this simple formula may help you focus on the positive and cope somewhat better.

A Accept—keep active and occupied.

D Direct yourself outward.

A Aim for reasonable goals and learn to completely relax.

P Pace your activities, staying within your limitations. (It may be necessary to reassess your priorities.)

T Take medications wisely. Be open and reasonable in dealing with your doctors.

Reprinted with permission of Chronic Pain Outreach of Greater St. Louis, Inc., (314) 768-1350.

Same Stimulus, Different Response

❖ When your pain is associated with something beneficial, such as in childbirth or winning a game, it's not accompanied by much anxiety, and suffering is minimized. There are many stories of injured athletes who finished an event, only to collapse in pain afterward.

❖ Patients who communicate openly with their physicians require less pain medication. This sense of relief seems to come from a reduction in psychological tension.

❖ Pain seems to be worse when the doctor is unavailable, like at night or during the weekend, and when you are alone or have nothing to keep your mind off the pain. Pain may astonishingly improve while you're on the way to see the doctor.

❖ The ability to tolerate pain is reduced with high anxiety, depression, an introverted personality, concentrating a lot on bodily functions, and focusing on the internal stimuli from your body. The ability to tolerate pain is increased with low anxiety, an extroverted personality, minimal concentration on your bodily functions, and focusing on external stimuli.

❖ Pain may be easier to control if you can deal with any anxiety and stay in touch with stimuli from the outside world. It helps if you know what the pain means and if you can provide a means of relief, whether it involves heat, traction, bracing, mechanical devices, cold, massage, relaxation techniques, imagery, pain medication, exercise, diversion, family and cultural dynamics, or your own unique personality and belief system.

From *Successful Living with Chronic Illness,* by Kathleen Lewis. © 1989. Avery Publishing Group, Garden City Park, NY $10. To order: (404) 491-6850.

Medication 101

There are several important points to remember about medication and pain control:

❖ **The medication must equal the pain.** Taking a drug designed for mild pain when you are experiencing severe pain is like using a squirt gun on a house fire. Be honest and specific about the degree of your pain. Otherwise, the prescribed drug may be inappropriate.

❖ **Medication must be taken before the pain becomes intense.** Many people "tough it out" and wait until the pain gets really bad before taking medication. Don't. For most people, it's best to take medication on a regular schedule (every three or four hours, for example) around the clock to prevent the pain cycle from starting.

❖ **Morphine is no longer considered a "last effort" drug.** The American College of Physicians, the American Medical Association, and the World Health Organization all agree that oral morphine is

the drug of choice for chronic severe pain. It's a myth that morphine use leads to addiction. When pain becomes less severe, your
need for the drug automatically decreases.

✧ **In short, the right drug in the right dose given at the right time
relieves 85 to 90 percent of pain.** People who are knowledgeable
about their pain and assertive enough to ask for what they need
usually achieve an acceptable level of pain control over long periods of time.

From *I Can Cope,* by Judith L. Johnson, RN, PhD, and Linda Klein. © 1994.
Chronimed Publishing, Minneapolis, MN $12.95.

Pain Down the Drain

STEP ONE

Allow yourself at least five minutes for this exercise. Get into the most comfortable position possible and close your eyes. Clear away any extraneous thoughts that might be interfering. You're going to use your imagination as if it were a television set, picturing your body.

STEP TWO

Imagine you are transparent and filled to the top of your head with green fluid (or any color that represents pain to you). Imagine the liquid beginning to drain out through your fingertips and toes. Picture the level of fluid beginning to drop, from the top of your head, past your eyes, nose, mouth, down through and out your fingertips. Feel the pain and tension draining from your body with the colored liquid. Let the liquid drain down past your back, hips, thighs, knees, legs, into your feet, and out the ends of your toes. (Perform this exercise slowly; don't try to rush.)

Now, picture your body and see if there are any puddles of pain left. If there are, imagine soaking them up with a paper towel.

STEP THREE
Finish your exercise by using the breathing technique on page XX for 30 seconds. Open your eyes; feel refreshed and relaxed.

From *Power Over Your Pain Without Drugs,* by Neal Olshan. © 1980. Beaufort Books/ SBN Publishing, New York, NY $12.95. (212) 727-0190.

Calming Pain Down

STEP ONE

When you first feel pain, don't panic. If you panic, the pain will probably increase. Panic and tension tend to increase pain.

STEP TWO

Don't let fear get the best of you. Calmly assess the situation. Be aware of where the pain is located, whether it is new or old, and how severe it is. Try not to let your imagination get the best of you.

STEP THREE

Inhale deeply through your nose. Try to take the air all the way down into your stomach and expand your stomach to fill your lungs completely. Exhale slowly through your mouth, trying to empty your lungs and stomach completely. As you exhale, your stomach should contract. Relax, and repeat twice.

Now inhale slowly through your nose to the count of two. Hold your breath to the count of three, and exhale through your mouth to the count of two. Relax to the count of four. Repeat this pattern for several minutes.

STEP FOUR

Get into the most comfortable position possible and close your eyes. Take a deep breath. Hold it for a count of three and let it out slowly for a count of three. Take another deep breath (count of three). Do this five times, and on the fifth deep breath, as you inhale, repeat to yourself the words "I am." Hold the deep breath for a brief count of two or three, and as you exhale, say to yourself, "pain-free." The repetition of the words "I am...pain-free" in sequence with your breathing will immediately counteract the fear or panic that generally starts at the onset of pain.

From *Power Over Your Pain Without Drugs,* by Neal Olshan. © 1980. Beaufort Books/ SBN Publishing, New York, NY $12.95. (212) 727-0190.

Alternative Routes

Although medicating pain is always an option, you may want to ask your doctor about these alternative approaches to pain control.

Behavioral Therapy: Biofeedback, relaxation training, or stress-management programs are often used to relieve pain, reduce muscle spasms, and diminish stress.

Transcutaneous Nerve Stimulation (TENS): TENS is a small battery-operated device that blocks out pain by delivering nonpainful electrical impulses to nerve fibers through the skin.

Acupuncture: As an alternative to TENS, electrical stimulation of acupuncture points is sometimes performed.

Rehabilitation Services: Physical and occupational therapy treatments may include exercise, whirlpool, ultrasound, massage, and manipulation.

Nerve Blocks: an injection of local anesthetic, with or without corti-sone-like medicines, around nerves or into joints. These may act to reduce swelling, irritation, muscle spasms, or abnormal nerve trans-missions that can cause pain.

Cryoanalgesia: freezing the affected area to reduce pain. Normally, it is used for pain generated from the chest wall.

Implantable Analgesia: time-released mechanism for releasing pain-relieving medication. The implant will deliver minimal amounts of pain-relieving medication into the spinal cord. Implantable epidural stimulators are also available for blocking lower-body pain.

Adapted from West County Pain Control Center, St. Louis, MO. (314) 567-0402 and the Pain Management Center, Christian Hospital Northeast, St. Louis, MO. (314) 355-2500, ext. 2500.

Healthstyles of the Rich and Famous

✦ Franklin Roosevelt led the nation and vigorously pursued wartime victory while confined to a wheelchair following adult-onset polio.

✦ Barbara Jordan, the Texas congresswoman, served the public well despite being in a wheelchair because of a neuromuscular disease.

✦ John Kennedy campaigned for the presidency and served in that office with often intense chronic pain as a result of a back injury.

✦ Beethoven wrote his final works as his hearing faded and ultimately deserted him.

✦ The astrophysicist Stephen Hawking wrote his best-selling *On the Origins of the Universe* while paralyzed by a neurological disease.

✧ Elizabeth Browning, bedridden with a back injury, wrote enduring romantic poetry from her sickroom.

✧ Florence Nightingale's disabling lung disease didn't stop her from giving advice on how to set up wartime medical services.

✧ Proust wrote under the stress of a disabling respiratory disease.

✧ Robert Louis Stevenson gave us the pleasure of his adventure novels written from the confines of his sickbed.

✧ Martha Graham, with severe arthritis, brought joy to millions with her innovative dance choreography.

✧ And Mickey Mantle slugged 536 home runs, despite the intense chronic pain and discomfort of injured and battered knees.

From _Healing the Body Betrayed: A Self-Paced, Self-Help Guide to Regaining Psychological Control of Your Chronic Illness,_ by Robert A. Klein, PhD, and Marcia Goodman Landau, PhD © 1992. Chronimed Publishing, Minneapolis, MN $12.95.

Mind Journeys

The Arthritis Foundation suggests these "mental excursions" to help you relax.

✧ Light a candle and focus your attention on the flame for a few minutes. Then close your eyes and watch the image of the flame for a minute or two.

✧ Imagine a white cloud floating toward you. It wraps itself around your pain and stress. Then a breeze comes. It blows away the cloud, taking your pain and stress with it.

✧ Think about a place you've been where you once felt pleasure and comfort. Imagine as much detail as possible—how it looks, smells, sounds, and feels. Recapture the positive feelings you had then and keep them in your mind. Don't make any room for negative thoughts, stress, or pain.

✧ Imagine that you've put all your concerns, worries, and pain in a helium-filled balloon. Now let go of the balloon and watch it float away.

Role Reversal

This visualization exercise is designed to help you "flip" the negative images you associate with your pain, tension, or discomfort into healing images. Make use of all your senses, since they're extremely powerful.

Ask yourself the following questions:

✧ If I were to draw a picture of my pain, associating it with some object or condition, what would that picture be?

✧ Is there a sound connected with the problem or pain? A grinding, perhaps, or gurgling?

✧ Is there a texture associated with it? A sore throat, for instance, might feel like sandpaper; an upset stomach might feel slimy.

✧ Is there a temperature associated with it? A headache might feel hot; a broken limb might feel cold.

✧ Is there a smell or taste associated with it?

✧ Is there a movement associated with it—churning, stabbing, pounding?

Now, "flip" these images. The essential consideration is what the problem or pain will look, feel, smell, sound, and taste like when it is alleviated or cured. For each image you formed in answering the previous questions, you'll now substitute its opposite.

As you relax, substitute a positive, healing image for each negative, painful one. Use words, if necessary, to reinforce this. Post a sign or note near you to remind yourself to flip often into a new set of images.

From *The Fine Art of Recuperation: Surviving and Thriving After Illness, Accident and Surgery,* by Regina Sara Ryan. © 1989, renewed 1997. Used with permission. For information contact: Hohm Press, PO Box 2501, Prescott, AZ 86302. 1-800-381-2700.

Interview Skills

Carry on a conversation with your pain or write out a dialogue with it in a journal. Ask your pain why it's here now, what it has to teach you, and how it can be alleviated.

part five

IMAGE CONSCIOUS

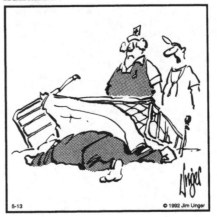

"Not the whole bed, nurse, just his mattress."

Follow the Bouncing Ball

First, close your eyes and relax. Think of a red ball, floating in a blue sky. Change the color of the ball. Move the ball from left to right, up and down; move the ball from side to side, back and forth.

Bring the ball closer to you. Then send it spinning away to the horizon, so far away you can't see it anymore. Then bring it back to you.

Turn the ball into a balloon, then into a kite. Change the kite into a bird, then into a ball again. Now, give up control of the image. Let your mind take the ball and do whatever it wants to with it.

Take control of the ball again. Bounce the ball through the sky. When you're ready to stop, open your eyes and restart your conscious mind.

From *You Can Relieve Pain: How Guided Imagery Can Help You Reduce Pain or Eliminate It Altogether,* by Ken Dachman and John Lyons. © 1990. HarperCollins, New York, NY $18.95. (212) 207-7000.

Daydream Believer

Close your eyes and imagine a favorite street, restaurant, movie theater, department store, or park. Think about what you would do in each place. Plan what you would wear and how you would get there, and imagine the sounds of each place. Daydreaming is total concentration and a way to temporarily experience being out of bed.

Sky Watching

If you're close to a window or can go outdoors, use the day or night sky as a source of meditation. Observe where your thoughts take you. Don't restrict your thoughts. Give them the whole sky to play in.

From *The Fine Art of Recuperation: Surviving and Thriving After Illness, Accident and Surgery,* by Regina Sara Ryan. © 1989, renewed 1997. Used with permission. For information contact: Hohm Press, PO Box 2501, Prescott, AZ 86302. 1-800-381-2700.

Palm Balm

This simple relaxation technique uses breathing, visualizing, and blocking sensory stimulation to the eyes.

1. Rub your palms together to warm them.

2. Place one cupped palm over each eye, the fingers of one hand crossing the fingers of the other hand on your forehead.

3. Keep your eyes open. Arrange your palms so no light can be seen.

4. Breathe softly and deeply for eight breaths, feeling a sense of warmth rising in your arms and hands, and bathing your eyes.

5. At the same time, imagine a happy and peaceful scene from your past.

6. After the eight breaths, remove your hands from your eyes and look softly around the room.

Staying Neutral

It can be difficult to relax when your mind and body are both clamoring for your attention with negative messages. One way to get around this is to concentrate on something that is neutral—neither good nor bad. This can help to clear the mind of the concerns of the moment, freeing it for more relaxing activity.

From *Coping With Pain: Focus on Cancer.* Vol. 1, No. 3, Spring 1991. The KSF Group, 630 Ninth Avenue, Suite 901, New York, NY 10036. (212) 582-5600.

Dive Into the Pool of Forgiveness

1. Close your eyes and begin to feel a sense of peace and stillness.

2. Take a few deep breaths. As you breathe out, imagine you are breathing out all tensions and thoughts. Breathe as deeply as you can.

3. As you breathe in, tell yourself you are breathing in peace and stillness. Continue to breathe in peace and breathe out negativity.

4. Imagine that in front of you is a pool of pure light.

5. As you imagine the pool, think of some of the things you would like to let go. They may be things about yourself or someone else.

6. Start to let go of these thoughts and feelings, releasing them into the pool. Breathe them out.

From *Coping with Cancer: Making Sense of It All,* by Rachel Clyne. © 1989 Thorsons Publishing Group/HarperCollins Publishing, Wellingborough, England, and New York, NY (212) 207-7000.

Mental Vacations

Sometimes simply letting your mind wander or "go on vacation" will help reduce your stress. Here are a few delightful suggestions from the Arthritis Foundation:

✦ Watch as a sunset slowly turns into evening. Now count the stars.

✦ Take your shoes off and dig your toes into the grass.

✦ Sit in a park on a warm, sunny day and listen to the birds.

✦ Stare into the flickering flames of a welcoming fireplace.

✦ Take a virtual reality tour with a computer game or Web site.

*P*icture *T*his

Do you have a photograph of yourself taken during one of your peak periods of health and vitality? It's time to get it out and keep it around. If you don't think you've looked well for a long time, search magazines for shots of healthy people. Clip these photos out and put them where you can see them. Now envision yourself smiling back from those pictures.

Word Power

This exercise uses visualization to improve the power of words to convince your mind that you are healing.

1. Choose some strong words that evoke a sense of strength and healing in you. Choose words like *yes, alive,* and *healthy.*

2. Imagine the words on huge billboards all over the city, in neon lights on the side of a building, or maybe carved out of the rock on the side of a mountain.

3. Take a favorite word for each day, allowing your choice of word to be determined by what you feel you need that day.

4. Think of your word every chance you get throughout the day. See it often. Repeat the word or words to yourself as you go about your activities.

5. To reinforce this, write your word on several small cards or pieces of paper. Put them around where you will see them frequently. Each time you see them, remember your image of the word, say it to yourself, and really feel its power.

From *The Fine Art of Recuperation: Surviving and Thriving After Illness, Accident and Surgery*, by Regina Sara Ryan. © 1989, renewed 1997. Used with permission. For information contact: Hohm Press, PO Box 2501, Prescott, AZ 86302. 1-800-381-2700.

A Fond Glance Backwards

Remember the 10 happiest days of your life. What were they? And why? Dwell on each day for at least 15 minutes.

From *The Fine Art of Recuperation: Surviving and Thriving After Illness, Accident and Surgery*, by Regina Sara Ryan. © 1989, renewed 1997. Used with permission. For information contact: Hohm Press, PO Box 2501, Prescott, AZ 86302. 1-800-381-2700.

part six

HEALTH CARE LAND

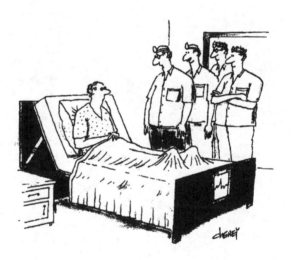

"Bob, these are doctors Burton, Kane, and Roycefield...
they'll be assisting me with your health insurance forms."

Tom Cheney ©1997 from The Cartoon Bank. All Rights Reserved.

The Missing Link

Many hospitals have an ombudsman or guest relations program that provides a specially trained representative who can run interference for you, respond to any special needs, or answer any questions. If the hospital does not offer this service, try the Social Work Department if you have a problem that cannot be straightened out.

That Touch of Home

If you're in the hospital or other alien surroundings, something old and familiar—something that looks and feels like home—will be a welcome emotional support: your own pajamas or nightgown, your own pillow and bedspread, those family photos, your coffee mug, your teddy bear, etc. Ask friends or family to help make your environment a place to heal, not just endure. Small comforts like these can make a tremendous difference in your ability to sustain the emotional ups and downs of this challenging time.

The New Patient Fuzzies

Feeling a little fuzzy during your first few hours in the hospital? It's natural and understandable. To help orient yourself, ask your nurse to write down the names of all the doctors and nurses who are treating you. Studies show that using someone's name can also help you get more personal attention and care.

From *Pregnancy Bedrest: A Guide for the Pregnant Woman and Her Family,* by Susan H. Johnston, M.S.W., and Deborah A. Kraut, M.I.L.R. © 1990 by Susan H. Johnston, and Deborah A. Kraut. Reprinted by permission of Henry Holt and Company, Inc.

Quiet on the Set!

One solution to the noise problem in hospitals is a pocket-size radio and tape player with a headset. That way you can drown out the offending sounds with pleasant tones of your own, whether it's your favorite music station or a stimulating talk show. Using high-density, soft earplugs, such as Flents Ear Stopples, is another solution. These and other types of earplugs are often sold at pharmacies or supermarkets.

*N*ursing *R*esources

It may not be apparent to you at first, but nurses are not just care-givers. They are prepared—assuming you ask them when they're not busy—to do all of the following:

✧ Explain the nature of your illness.

✧ Review the details of your treatment.

✧ Evaluate the side effects of treatment.

✧ Discuss your condition with your doctor.

✧ Give comfort to you and your family.

✧ Teach you how to care for your condition.

From *You Can Make It Back: Coping With Serious Illness,* by Paul M. Levitt and Elissa S. Guralnick. © 1985. Facts on File Publications, New York, NY $16.95. Currently out of print but still available in many libraries. (212) 683-2244.

Sock Strategies

An extra pair of socks can cover your cold hands or cold feet if the hospital is cool. Take several pairs along with you or ask a friend or relative to retrieve them if you forget. The nurse may also be able to provide you with a pair.

From *Successful Living With Chronic Illness*, by Kathleen Lewis. © 1989. Avery Publishing Group, Garden City Park, NY $10. To order: (404) 491-6850.

*A*lternate *V*iewpoints

Keep in mind that cooperation with your treatment does not mean blind obedience. If you disagree with your treatment plan, tell your doctor. If your doctor suggests a plan that is impractical for you, discuss it. Come to some understanding with each other. Usually, many more options are available than are immediately apparent. Explore alternatives. Accepting treatment recommendations passively and then resisting them actively is a waste of your time and effort.

From *The Fine Art of Recuperation: Surviving and Thriving After Illness, Accident and Surgery,* by Regina Sara Ryan. © 1989, renewed 1997. Used with permission. For information contact: Hohm Press, PO Box 2501, Prescott, AZ 86302. 1-800-381-2700.

Worth Studying

Even before you begin to be treated, you should study your medical insurance policy and meet with your company's benefits officer, or call the agent who sold you the plan, to determine what costs will be covered. You should know, for example, if your policy will pay for:

✧ unlimited hospitalization

✧ a private room (or the cost difference between a private and semi-private room)

✧ a private nurse

✧ doctor's fees

✧ therapy or psychiatric counseling

✧ rehabilitation

✧ home health care

✧ equipment—such as a dialysis unit—for use in the home

✧ cosmetic surgery for reconstruction or to change a limb or face
   altered by surgery or disease

✧ prosthetic limbs or body parts

✧ dental care

✧ prescription drugs

The more familiar you are with your policy's provisions, the more
information you can give your doctor that may affect your "bottom
line." Your doctor may be able to adjust your treatment plan to take
maximum advantage of your coverage.

From *You Can Make It Back: Coping With Serious Illness,* by Paul M. Levitt and Elissa S.
Guralnick. © 1985. Facts on File Publications, New York, NY $16.95. Currently out
of print but still available at many libraries. (212) 683-2244.

Active, Not Passive

People who are actively involved in their medical care do better than those who are passive. To find out if you and your doctor are communicating effectively, answer these five simple questions:

1. Does your doctor seem impatient or hurried when you start discussing your questions?

2. Do you abbreviate or rush your questions so you won't keep the doctor waiting when he or she has so many other people to see?

3. Are your questions met with vague, overly complex, or evasive answers?

4. Are you unable to explain to friends and family what your doctor told you?

5. Are you relieved to be able to turn to nurses, nurses' aides, or orderlies to explain things to you?

If the answer is yes to any of the above, try these phrases to enhance communication and understanding with your doctor:

✧ "Could you please explain that last part again?"

✧ "What are you really telling me I can expect next?"

✧ "I'd appreciate it if you could list my options for me."

✧ "Excuse me, doctor, but I think it would help me to have my (husband/wife/friend) here for this discussion, so I'd like to wait until they're here."

From *What Your Doctor Didn't Learn in Medical School...And What You Can Do About It,* by Stuart M. Berger, M.D. © 1988. William Morrow & Company, New York, NY $18.95. (212) 261-6500.

Dealing With Surgery

Here are some suggestions to help reduce the understandable anxieties surrounding surgery:

✧ Insist your doctor thoroughly explain the surgical procedure and everything that follows.

✧ Consider seeking a second opinion.

✧ Be frank in discussing your fears with the surgeon.

✧ Don't be disappointed if your surgeon's not warm and outgoing.

✧ Ask to meet the anesthesiologist.

✧ Treat the nurse who performs the preoperative workup as a valuable information resource.

From *You Can Make It Back: Coping With Serious Illness,* by Paul M. Levitt and Elissa S. Guralnick. © 1985. Facts on File Publications, New York, NY $16.95. Currently out of print but still available at many libraries. (212) 683-2244.

True Admissions

One of the most boring (and stressful) parts of a hospital stay occurs right at the beginning—getting admitted. This process can go smoothly, or it can be a nightmare. The purpose of admission is to take care of the paperwork for billing insurers, for billing you, and for the permanent medical record.

On a normal day, the admission process takes about 20 minutes. But if you phone ahead (in some hospitals they'll even call you) and give your insurance and personal information such as birth date and Social Security and insurance card numbers, you can often cut that time to about 10 minutes.

From "Your Guide to Getting Good Hospital Care," by Tim Friend. © *USA Today*, June 19, 1991. Reprinted with permission. $107 per year for 5 issues per week. (800) 872-0001.

Moving On

Professionals offer many tips for people who must leave the work force because of an illness or injury:

❖ Choose a doctor you like and rely on him or her for encouragement, not just prescriptions.

❖ Expect emotional changes. Seek counseling or develop a caring network by contacting support groups. (See the *Encyclopedia of Associations* at your library as a starting point.)

❖ Contact the local Center for Independent Living to obtain peer counseling and learn how to maintain your independence.

❖ Find out what insurance benefits your employer, union, or association provides.

✧ If applying for Social Security disability, contact the Social Security Administration for information. Also, try to manage the negative effects of the disability qualification process by mentally separating yourself from it. Remind yourself that nothing is meant to be a personal attack on you.

✧ Create a daily structure that includes exercise, particularly an aquatics program, walking, or a set of exercises designed for you.

✧ If at home, build a telephone network with peers, friends, and relatives. Also, continue socializing by inviting friends over for a potluck dinner once a month. (You could ask each guest to bring food and a guest you don't know.)

✧ Consider going back to school via TV correspondence courses or the Internet.

From *Arthritis Today: The Magazine of Help and Hope.* September-October 1990. 1314 Spring St. N.W., Atlanta, GA 30309. The magazine is available free to those who join the Arthritis Foundation. (404) 872-7100.

part seven

VISITING OURS

HERMAN®

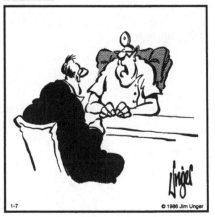

1-7   © 1986 Jim Unger

"You need more exercise. Go and get me a cheeseburger with onions."

Helping Hands

If friends offer to help you, don't be shy about telling them the things that would make you feel better right now. If you can't think of anything, you might ask them to bring over dinner the first night you're home from the hospital.

From Ellen Bern and Barry Mizes, St. Louis, MO.

Count Your Supporters

It can be very helpful to take a few minutes to remember the people who could assist you now or at some later time. This exercise can help:

1. Divide a piece of paper into two columns. On the top of the left-hand column, write "Places I go." On the top of the right-hand column, write "People I meet."

2. Start by listing all the places you go to or went to regularly before your accident or illness. Include evening places as well as daytime places, places you go once a month, like a meeting or your church or social group, and even places you go infrequently, as with that annual visit to see your childhood friend.

3. On the right side of the chart, list the people you regularly see or meet at the places you have indicated.

4. Now take a fresh sheet to continue your list of contacts. Write the name of anyone you know who meets the following criteria.

trustworthy with money	very good listener
understanding and compassionate	seems to enjoy helping others
easy to be with	makes me laugh
very bright about practical matters	offered help if I ever needed it

Just in case you've forgotten someone obvious, make a list of friends, colleagues at work, and relatives.

5. Put a check or asterisk next to the names of the people you would be comfortable either sharing with or asking for some help. Double the symbol for those you feel very comfortable about, and you'll have your first-string support list.

From *The Fine Art of Recuperation: Surviving and Thriving After Illness, Accident and Surgery,* by Regina Sara Ryan. © 1989, renewed 1997. Used with permission. For information contact: Hohm Press, PO Box 2501, Prescott, AZ 86302. 1-800-381-2700.

Healing Hugs

Sometimes a good hug is all you need to make your day. Yet many folks don't give themselves permission to hug or hold in a way that really allows for a merging of life-energy. A healing hug is one that allows you to relax into another's arms, if only for a few seconds, to feel the tangible, physical support of another human being. You might suggest that your friend or caregiver give you a "breakfast hug," my term for a gentle but complete embrace in which one partner acts as the warm toast, the other partner as the butter. Maintain the contact until both of you agree the butter is completely melted, absorbed into the toast.

From *The Fine Art of Recuperation: Surviving and Thriving After Illness, Accident and Surgery,* by Regina Sara Ryan. © 1989, renewed 1997. Used with permission. For information contact: Hohm Press, PO Box 2501, Prescott, AZ 86302. 1-800-381-2700.

*T*ough *T*opics

If you're having trouble talking about your illness or injury with people close to you, here are some opening statements for initiating discussion, adapted from *The Road Back to Health,* by Neil Fiore, PhD.

◇ I feel like my illness/injury has come between us, and I'm becoming isolated and alienated from you. We're both suffering privately. Is there anything I can do to help you through this time?

◇ We've been dancing around the issue of my condition a lot lately. Can't we find a way to really talk?

◇ It's hard for me to tell you my feelings about my illness/injury. And I'm afraid it will upset you if I bring it up.

From *I Can Cope* by Judith L. Johnson, R.N., PhD, and Linda Klein © 1994. Chronimed Publishing, Minneapolis, MN $12.95.

Just Visiting

If you're scared, lonely, or worried about tomorrow's procedure, then it's your right as a patient and as a fragile human being toohave your visitor or visitors stay with you past visiting hours. Perhaps you need your visitor to spend the night nearby. If the nurse tries to send the visitor away, stand your ground. Ask to see the head nurse. If you're not satisfied, demand to see the patient's representative or the hospital administrator, no matter what time it is. If you must, call your doctor at home. You can have somebody there with you past hours if you want. On the other hand, if you do not want visitors, politely ask the staff for their support in keeping visitors away.

Holiday Strategies

Holidays have a way of heightening our emotions. The highs and lows of happiness and depression, and blessings and losses are all magnified. We are thankful for the blessings of love and remembrance. We also become sad as we are vividly reminded of losses—health, goals, ambitions, functions—maybe even loved ones or changed relationships. It can be a sober time for reflection. You might take some time to think about where your life is and what is really important.

Try not to spend your holidays completely alone if you can help it. It's very important to share them with someone else. Find someone to spend a little time with, even if it's just on the phone. Find your own unique way to reach out to others, staying within your limits.

From *Successful Living with Chronic Illness,* by Kathleen Lewis. © 1989. Avery Publishing Group, Garden City Park, NY $10. To order: (404) 491-6850.

Talk It Out

Bottling up all the worries and fears you have right now only builds up tension. Someone once said a good friend is worth 100 psychiatrists. Confide in someone you respect and trust—your husband or wife, father or mother, a good friend, your clergyperson, your family physician, a teacher, or a school counselor. Talking about problems won't solve them. But just having the conversation will reduce stress. And then seek professional assistance if necessary. You're worth it!

From *I Can Cope,* by Judith L. Johnson, RN, PhD, and Linda Klein. © 1994. Chronimed Publishing, Minneapolis, MN $12.95.

$\mathcal{W}$elcome $\mathcal{S}$upport

Many pain outreach programs offer regular monthly meetings, a 24-hour a day answering service, a resource library, newsletters, and ongoing educational presentations. To get information about local chapters, call or write:

National Chronic Pain Outreach, 7979 Old Georgetown Rd., Suite 100, Bethesda, MD 20814-2429. Phone (301) 652-4948. Or fax (301) 907-0745.

American Chronic Pain Association, P.O. Box 850, Rocklin, CA 95677. Phone (916) 632-0922.

Reprinted with permission of Chronic Pain Outreach of Greater St. Louis, Inc., (314) 768-1350.

The Leaning Tower of Strength

Learn to lean on people—not a lot, but just enough to let them know you're there.

part eight

EDIBLY YOURS

HERMAN®

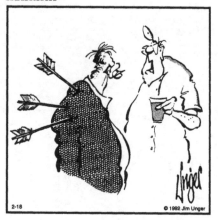

"Drink this, but stand over there by the sink."

"Dry Mouth" Help

If NPO (nothing by mouth) is written on your chart and you have dry mouth as a result, here are some helpful suggestions to follow once you get your doctor's or nurse's OK:

❖ Rinse your mouth with mouthwash or brush your teeth, being careful not to swallow.

❖ Suck a slightly damp, clean washcloth, letting dry mucous membranes absorb the moisture.

❖ Keep lips moistened with lip balm.

❖ Drink plenty of fluids right up to the time the NPO begins.

❖ Ask for a vaporizer.

From *Successful Living with Chronic Illness,* by Kathleen Lewis. © 1989. Avery Publishing Group, Garden City Park, NY $10. To order: (404) 491-6850.

The Mood for Food

Even when you start feeling better after an accident or injury, food may still not sound appealing. Many people have found the following techniques make eating easier and more enjoyable:

✧ Create the right atmosphere. Set the table with place mats and flowers. Play pleasant dinner music, and perhaps invite family and friends to join you. You'll be more relaxed and you may discover you are more hungry than you thought.

✧ With your doctor's approval, have a glass of wine or beer before a meal. It's relaxing and can also be an appetite stimulant. Good odors may help, too. The smell of a fresh loaf of bread or cake baking can make you hungry for those foods.

✧ Take advantage of the "up" times. Eat well when you're feeling good. This is also a good time to prepare meals that can be frozen and easily reheated on your more difficult days.

✧ Use paper plates, paper napkins, and disposable silverware as often as possible to save on dishwashing. Use disposable pans for cooking (foil containers from frozen dinners work well).

✧ Eat small, frequent meals. Instead of planning on three meals a day, eat just a little bit at a time, but more often.

✧ Keep snacks on hand. Good ideas for easy snacks are ice cream, peanut butter and crackers, pudding, peanuts, dried fruits, and canned milk shakes.

✧ Eat solid foods before liquids. Liquids may fill you up before you have met your nutritional needs. Save them for after the meal.

From *I Can Cope,* by Judith L. Johnson, RN, PhD, and Linda Klein. © 1994. Chronimed Publishing, Minneapolis, MN $12.95.

Urination Inspiration

One of the most common postsurgical side effects of general anesthesia is difficulty or inability urinating. To "inspire" your body back to normal, hold your hand under warm running water while sitting on the toilet. If you use a bedpan, put one hand in a basin of warm water on a bedside table and move your hand around slowly.

Sweet Rx

Chocolate contains phenylethylamine, the same chemical the brain produces when people fall in love. The chemical causes a happy, slightly dreamy feeling by stepping up the heart rate and the body's energy level.

So, if you don't have a health problem such as high cholesterol or diabetes, and if you're not on a low-fat or caffeine-free diet, you may want to ask your doctor if it's OK for you to indulge in this natural mood elevator.

Printed in the USA
CPSIA information can be obtained
at www.ICGtesting.com
JSHW082208140824
68134JS00014B/507

9 780471 346531